Diverticular Diseases *and* Diverticulitis Diet

Diverticulitis Cause, Symptoms, Diet, Treatment & Prevention

ALICIA DENNIS

1

monetary loss due to the information herein, either directly or indirectly.

Respective authors own all copyrights not held by the publisher. The information herein is offered for informational purposes solely, and is universal as so. The presentation of the information is without contract or any type of guarantee assurance.

The trademarks that are used are without any consent, and the publication of the trademark is without permission or backing by the trademark owner. All trademarks and brands within this book are for clarifying purposes only and are the owned by the owners themselves, not affiliated with this document.

Contents

Introduction

I Want to thank you and congratulate you for downloading the book, "**Diverticular Diseases** *and* **Diverticulitis Diet:** *Diverticulitis Cause, Symptoms, Diet, Treatment & Prevention*".

This book contains demonstrated strides and techniques on the most proficient method to beat Diverticular malady and to forestall it through enhancing your eating routine.

Diverticulitis influences the lives of numerous Americans and it is absolutely preventable with a couple of basic changes in eating regimen. Regardless of the fact that the infection has created, with an enhanced eating routine the side effects can be decreased and a man can keep on living a solid life. Much appreciated again to download this book, I trust you appreciate it!

Chapter 1

Diverticulitis (Diverticulosis, Diverticular Disease)

In our society today there are many things that all people know they have to be careful about. Their cholesterol counts are easy to find out as are the readings of their blood pressure. Is there too much salt in your diet? Of course we are all well aware of these issues but ask anyone about Diverticular disease and most likely it will be followed by a blank stare. Even though diverticulitis is a very common disease, few people have any idea exactly what the disease actually is and better yet how it can be prevented.

It is a fact that about 1 in 3 people suffer from the problem of diverticulosis, yet since it has very few symptoms it is never recognized until it develops into a case of diverticulitis. Then the symptoms are very painful and noticeable and it can affect your life. The best part of this is that the disease can be completely avoided if a person makes an effort to concentrate on their diet and eat a bit better in their lives.

Diverticulosis and diverticulitis definition and facts

A great many people with diverticulosis (Diverticular illness) have few or no side effects; in any case, indications that can happen with diverticulosis, which then might be called **"Diverticular disease"** incorporate Stomach pain, Constipation, and Diarrhea.

At the point when diverticulosis is connected with irritation and infection it is called "diverticulitis."

Diverticulitis and Diverticular disease can be determined to have barium X-beams, sigmoidoscopy, colonoscopy, or CT scan.

Treatment of diverticulitis and Diverticular infection can incorporate high fiber eating diet, and anti-spasmodic drugs.

Foods to eat that may avoid diverticulitis flares incorporate foods grown from the ground, vegetables, and whole grains.

It has been proposed that individuals with diverticulitis abstain from eating seeds, nuts, and corn; be that as it may, there is little confirmation to support this suggestion.

At the point when diverticulosis is connected with aggravation and disease the condition is called diverticulitis.

Complexities of diverticulosis and diverticulitis incorporate rectal bleeding, stomach infections, and colon hindrance

What is diverticulosis?

The colon (internal organ or huge inside) is a long tube-like structure roughly 6 feet long that stores and afterward wipes out waste material left over after processing of sustenance in the small digestive tract happens. It is imagined that weight inside the colon causes protruding pockets of tissue (sacs) that push out from the colonic dividers as a man ages. A little swelling sac pushing outward from the colon wall is called a diverticulum.

More than one protruding sac is alluded to in the plural as Diverticular.

Diverticular can happen all through the colon however are most basic close to the end of the left colon, alluded to as the sigmoid colon, in Western nations. In Asia, the Diverticular happen for the most part on the right half of the colon. The state of having this Diverticular in the colon is called diverticulosis.

Diverticular are regular in the Western world yet are uncommon in ranges, for example, Asia and Africa. Diverticular increment with age. They are remarkable before the age of 40, yet are found in more than 74% of individuals beyond 80 years old years in the U.S. A man with diverticulosis typically has few or no side effects. The most well-known symptoms connected with diverticulosis are stomach pain, blockage, and loose bowels.

In some of these patients the side effects might be because of the associative nearness of bad tempered inside disorder (IBS) or variations from the norm in the capacity of the muscles of the sigmoid colon (in which case it is alluded to as Diverticular disease); basic Diverticular ought to bring about no symptoms. Every so often, bleeding starts from a diverticulum, and it is alluded to as Diverticular bleeding.

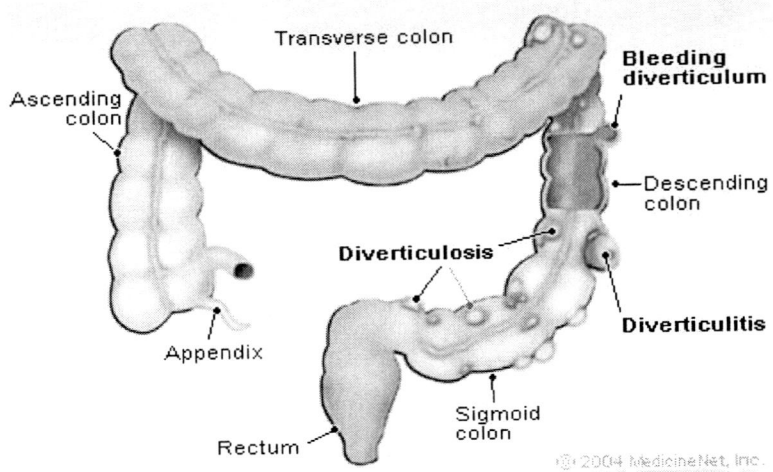

Transverse colon

Bleeding
diverticulum

Ascending
colon

Descending
colon

Diverticulosis

Diverticulitis

Appendix

Sigmoid
colon

Rectum

© 2004 MedicineNet, Inc.

Diverticular Disease

What is diverticulitis?

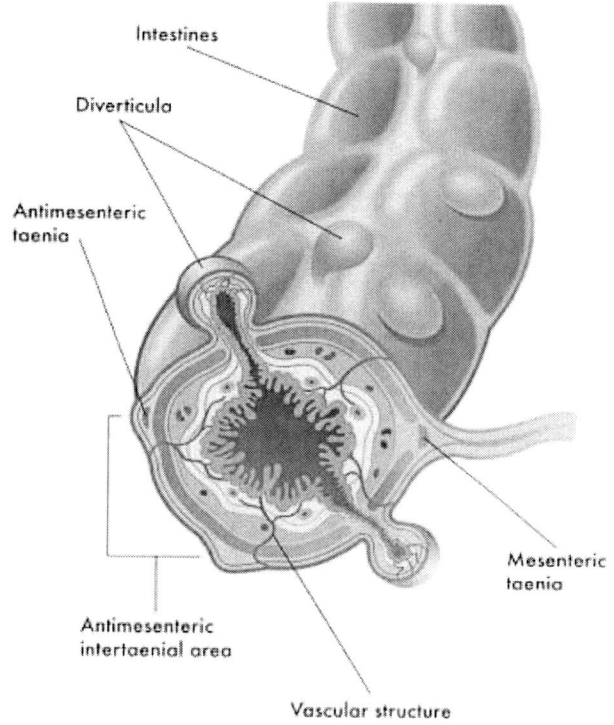

At the point when a diverticulum breaks and contamination sets in around the diverticulum, the condition is called diverticulitis. An individual experiencing diverticulitis regularly has stomach torment, stomach delicacy, colonic check, and a raised white platelet number in the blood, and fever.

What causes Diverticular and how do Diverticular structure?

The strong mass of the colon becomes thicker with age, despite the fact that the reason for this thickening is unclear. It might mirror the expanding weights required by the colon to eliminate feces.

For instance, an eating routine low in fiber can prompt little, hard stools which are hard to pass and which require expanded weight to pass. The absence of fiber and little stools additionally may permit fragments of the colon to shut off from whatever is left of the colon when the colonic muscle in the portion contracts. The pressure in these shut off fragments may turn out to be high since the expanded weight can't disperse to whatever remains of the colon. After some time, high weights in the colon push the internal intestinal coating outward (herniation) through frail zones in the strong dividers. These pockets or sacs that create are called Diverticular.

Absence of fiber in the eating diet has been thought to be the in all likelihood reason for Diverticular, and there is a decent connection among social orders far and wide between the measure of fiber in the eating diet and the prevalence of Diverticular. In any case, examines have not discovered comparative connections amongst fiber and Diverticular inside individual social orders. Numerous individuals with Diverticular disease have unnecessary thickening of the solid mass of the colon where the Diverticular structure. The muscle additionally contracts all the more unequivocally. These irregularities of the muscle might contribute variables in the development of Diverticular. Microscopic examination of the edges of the Diverticular hint at irritation, and it has been proposed that aggravation might be essential for the arrangement of the Diverticular and not only the consequence of them

What are diverticulitis symptoms?

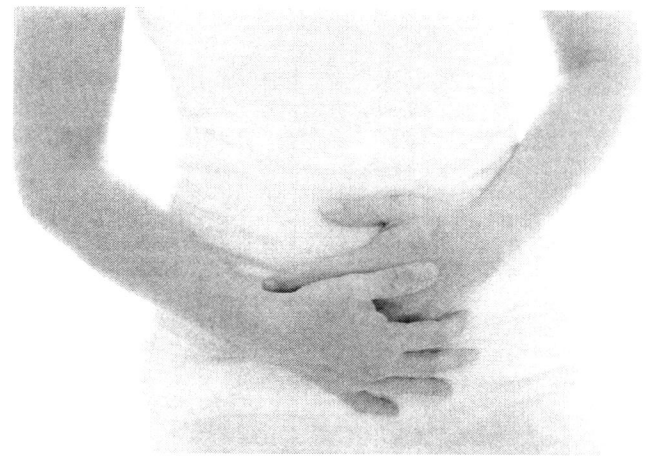

Most patients with diverticulosis have few or no symptoms. The diverticulosis in these people is discovered by the way during tests for other intestinal issues. It has been thought upwards of 20% of people with diverticulosis will create symptoms identified with the diverticulosis, essentially diverticulitis; nonetheless, the latest study recommends that the occurrence is more like 5%.

The most widely recognized signs and symptoms of diverticulitis include:

- Marked change in bowel habits
- Severe abdominal pain
- Cramping
- Tenderness in the lower abdomen
- Nausea
- Alternating diarrhea and constipation
- Fever and/or chills

Causes of Diverticulitis

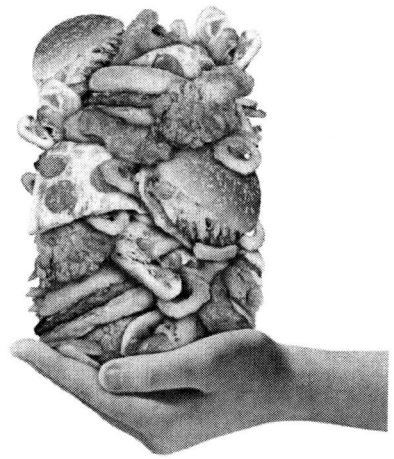

Today's ordinary western diet regularly comprises of exceedingly handled foods, sugar, and undesirable fats. This sort of diet adds to the advancement of Diverticular, and an infection.

Eating a diet rich with fiber can forestall diverticulitis, and aides in the recuperating of the colon. In addition a terrible eating routine, there are other danger elements to consider:

• Aging

• Obesity

- Smoking

- Prescription pharmaceuticals including sedatives, steroids, and non-steroidal anti-inflammatory

- Lack of customary high-impact exercise

These danger components, joined with a diet ailing in fundamental fiber, and high in creature fats, can prompt the advancement of marble-sized Diverticular in the digestive tract.

The subsequent aggravation, disease, and spillage into the stomach pit is uncomfortable, best case scenario, and can possibly bring about genuine intricacies

3 Natural Steps to Treat Diverticulitis
STEP 1: The Healing Diverticulitis Diet

STAGE 1

During a diverticulitis flare-up, or at first symptoms, it is critical to bail your digestive tract wipe itself out, and start to mend. Begin by utilizing my beef bone soup recipe.

Beef bone broth is a standout amongst the most mending foods you can expend. It's rich in supplements like gelatin and glycine, which secure and recuperate your broken gut, skin and digestive tract.

Beef Bone Broth Recipe
Total Time: 48 hours

Serves: Varies

INGREDIENTS:

- 4 pounds beef bones with marrow
- 4 carrots, chopped
- 4 celery stalks, chopped

- 2 medium onions, peel on, sliced in half lengthwise and quartered
- 4 garlic cloves, peel on and smashed
- 1 teaspoon kosher salt
- 1 teaspoon whole peppercorns
- 2 bay leaves
- 3 sprigs fresh thyme
- 5-6 sprigs parsley
- 1/4 cup ACV
- 18-20 cups cold water

DIRECTIONS:

1. Place all ingredients in a 10 quart capacity crock-pot.
2. Add in water.
3. Bring to a boil over high heat; reduce and simmer gently, skimming the fat that rises to the surface occasionally.
4. Simmer for 24-48 hours.
5. Remove from heat and allow to cool slightly.

6. Discard solids and strain remainder in a bowl through a colander. Let stock cool to room temperature, cover and chill.

7. Use within a week or freeze up to 3 months.

Eating bone soups produced using meat, chicken, sheep and fish recuperates broken gut disorder, enhances joint wellbeing, supports the resistant system, and even diminishes cellulite, all while helping to heal the digestive tract.

Bone broth with cooked vegetables and a little bit of meat, gives key supplements your body needs, including calcium, magnesium, phosphorus, silicon, sulfur, and that's just the beginning, in an effortlessly processed way.

You may add vegetables to your bone broth including carrots, celery and garlic or for variety, you may include an egg poachedin the stock. Furthermore, taste on warm ginger tea a few times every day to lessen aggravation and help in assimilation. Ginger is a healing food that helps your resistant and digestive systems.

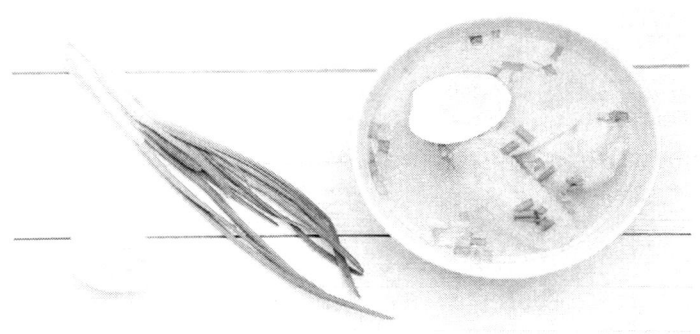

For beef, the collagen in the bones separates into gelatin inside around 48 hours, and for chicken it is around 24. You can make soup in less time, yet to get the most out of the bones, I suggest making it in a stewing pot more like 48 hours.

Gelatin has stunning curative properties and even helps people with food sensitivities and hypersensitivities endure these foods all the more effortlessly. It likewise advances probiotic parity, while separating proteins making them less demanding to process. Reality about probiotics and digestive issues is that they make a solid situation in your paunch. During this first period of the diverticulitis diet, devour just clear bone juices, clear crisp squeezes no ash), and calming ginger tea.

STAGE 2

Once the diverticulitis symptoms have facilitated, you can proceed onward to stage two of the diverticulitis diet and present effectively edible foods including ground, steamed and after that pureed products of the soil, while as yet drinking ginger tea and bone broth soups.

Juicing new natural foods grown from the ground can give a support of supplements. Carrots, beets, grapes, apples, lettuce and watercress can be juiced and appreciated during this stage. Maintain a strategic distance from foods with extreme skins and little seeds as they can aggregate in Diverticular sacs.

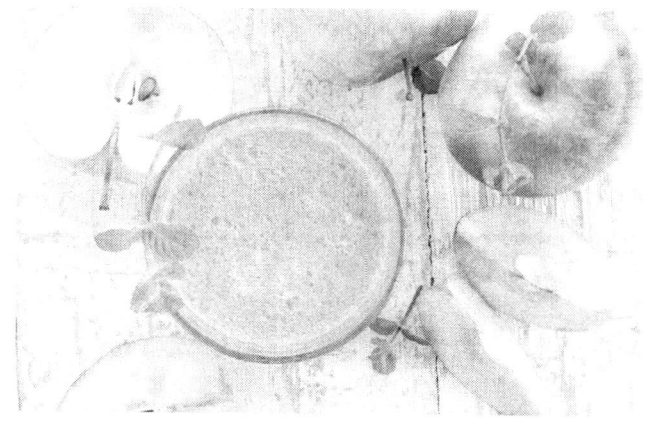

STAGE 3

At the point when your body has adjusted to the foods in Stage 2, begin to include fiber rich foods including crude products of the soil, and grungy grains, for example, quinoa, dark rice, matured grains, or sprouted lentils. It is essential to avoid entire nuts and seeds, as they can without much of a stretch get to be caught in the Diverticular, eating additional harm.

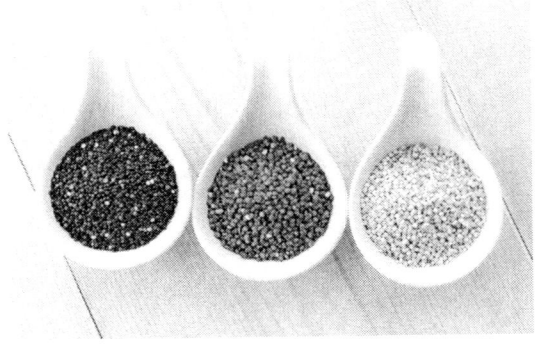

While seeds, nuts and popcorn are not the reason for diverticulitis, during this phase in healing, it is best to maintain a strategic distance from them. Once your diverticulitis symptoms have ebbed, you can come back to getting a charge out of these foods, and others, with some restraint.

Listen to your body; if anytime you begin to experience diverticulitis symptoms once more, come back to the past stage. It might take the length of a couple of months to totally recuperate your digestive tract.

STAGE 4

As indicated by analysts at the University of Oxford, fiber reduces the danger of Diverticular disease. The study concentrated on fiber from natural products, vegetables, oats, and potatoes.

So over the initial few days of stage four, present high-fiber foods bit by bit, including only one new nourishment each 3-4 days.

As your body adjusts you can start devouring around 25-35 grams of fiber every day, to fight off any potential flare-ups, while your digestive tract mends. Include a few potatoes, sweet potatoes, root vegetables, then gradually attempt some non-prepared grains/beans, for example, oats or lentils.

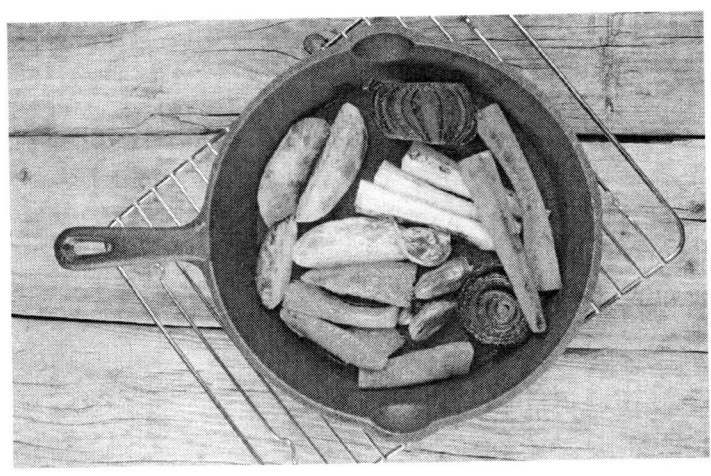

One important qualification is the contrast between solvent fiber, and insoluble fiber. Dissolvable fiber really holds water, and transforms into a gel during the digestive procedure. The gel moderates the processing, considering more prominent assimilation of key supplements. Insoluble fiber, then again, adds mass to stools, permitting foods to all the more rapidly leave your system.

Foods high in dissolvable fiber incorporate oat grain, nuts, seeds, beans, lentils grain, and peas. Insoluble fiber is found in foods including entire grains, wheat grain, and vegetables.

Scientists at the Department of Nutrition at Harvard Medical School found that it is the insoluble fiber that declines hazard for creating Diverticular disease. Be that as it may, don't let this influence you from eating an adjusted diet. You don't need to wipe out dissolvable fiber, nor if you.

Keeping up a sound parity of protein, fiber, and crisp leafy foods, is key for keeping diverticulitis from erupting.

STEP 2. *Supplements to Treat Diverticulitis*

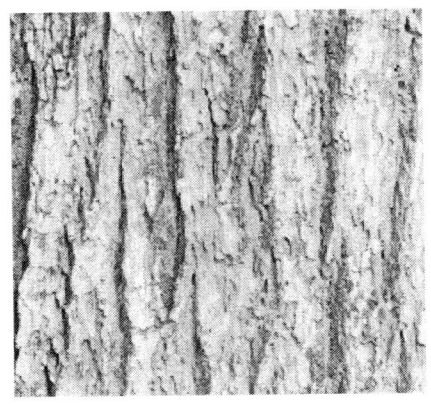

SLIPPERY ELM

Local Americans have utilized dangerous elm for quite a long time both remotely, and inside to soothe digestive issues and relieve coughs and sore throats.

Today, it is prescribed to relieve the symptoms of GERD, Crohn's disease, IBS, and digestive miracle. Begin by taking 500 milligrams, 3 times day by day, over the span of the diverticulitis diet. Make sure to take with a full glass of water, or other clear fluid.

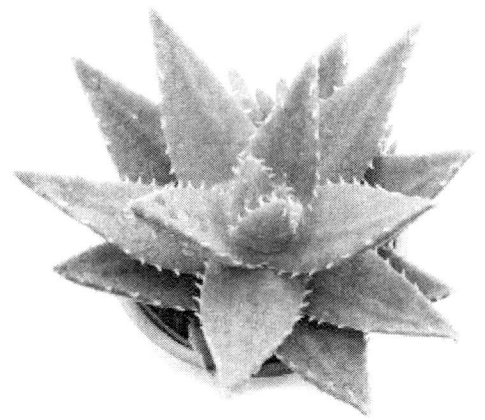

ALOE

Aloe, in a juice form, helps in absorption, standardizes pH levels, regularizes bowel handling, and energizes sound digestive microorganisms. It is important to maintain a strategic distance from aloe Vera juice with "aloe latex", as it can cause severe stomach cramping and diarrhea.

12 to 16 ounces for each day of aloe juice is prescribed; any more than that can advance aggravate your system.

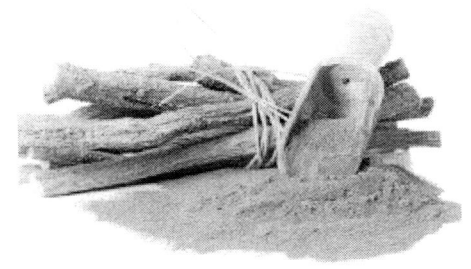

LICORICE ROOT

Licorice Root brings down stomach acid levels, can relieve acid reflux, and goes about as a mild laxative to clear your colon of waste. This root expands bile, supporting in absorption, while bringing down cholesterol levels. Take 100 milligrams every day while encountering diverticulitis symptoms.

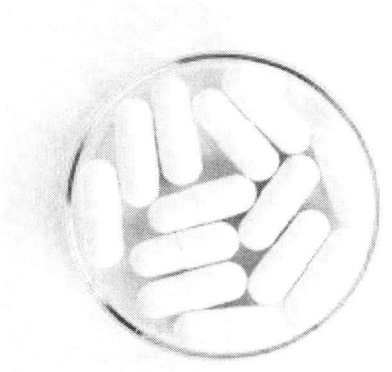

DIGESTIVE ENZMES

In addition to healing your colon from diverticulitis, the general objective of the diverticulitis diet, supplements, and way of life changes, is to urge your digestive tract to work ideally.

Digestive enzymes separate foods, making it conceivable to assimilate supplements. People with assimilation issues can take digestive supplements that contain crucial catalysts to encourage absorption.

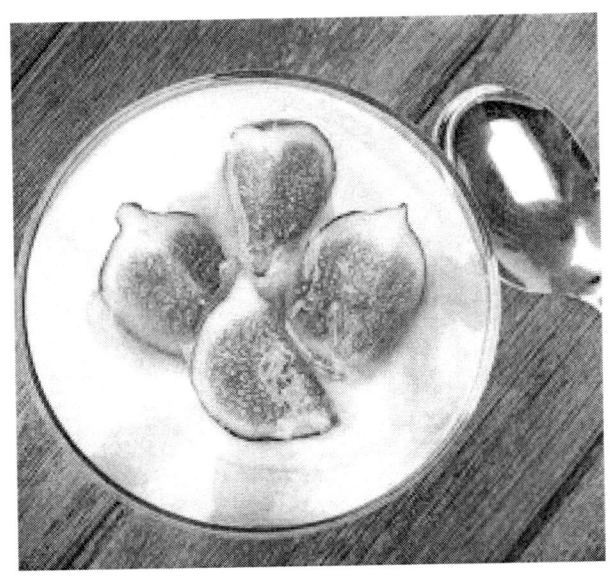

PROBIOTICS

Live probiotics ought to be added to the diet to invalidate food sensitivities, and ease digestive upset including blockage, gas, and bloating. Probiotics are sound microscopic organisms that generally line your digestive tract to battle disease. On the off chance that you have diverticulitis you require an influx of these microorganisms to help in the healing of your colon, while preventing disease repeat.

STEP 3. . *Way of life Changes Necessary to Treat Diverticulitis*

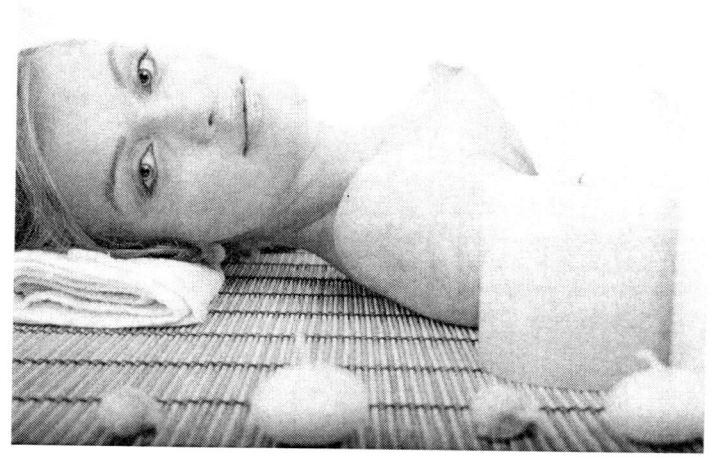

Diverticulitis requires more than only a recuperating diverticulitis diet, and supplements to help in a solid digestive tract. Digestion begins in the mouth. It is important to completely bite every chomp of food, until it is about condensed. The more you separate the food before it hits the stomach, the more prepared supplements are prepared to be ingested.

Medical studies demonstrate that the blend of physical action and high fiber diets avoids Diverticular disease. Running, or utilizing a rebounder every day, eases symptoms and decrease flare-ups. Indeed, even direct force exercise controls inside capacities, decreases push, and backings sound weight.

Your mental wellbeing is a necessary piece of your health; overseeing anxiety and learning powerful ways of dealing with stress is key. Stress influences the psyche, as well as the body also Straining while on the can makes an excess of weight in the colon bringing about little tears. Hoist feet somewhat on a stool as this decreases straining.

Diverticulitis diet: Foods to maintain a strategic distance from and foods that relieve symptoms once shaped, Diverticular don't leave; they are lasting. No treatment has been appeared to treat or counteract Diverticular disease or diverticulitis. In any case proposals have been made concerning which foods to eat, and which foods to avoid.

Foods to eat that may prevent flares

Since one hypothesis holds that it is decreased fiber in the diet that causes diverticulitis, diets high in fiber is the most suggested treatment for Diverticular. Fiber plainly expands stool mass and forestalls obstruction, and, on the off chance that it truly reduces pressures in the colon, hypothetically it might avert further Diverticular development or exacerbating of the Diverticular condition.

Foods high in fiber include:

Fruits and vegetables

Legumes/beans, (for example, Lima, kidney, cannellini, and red kidney beans; chickpeas, split peas, and tofu)

Whole grains (for example, brown rice, cracked wheat, oatmeal, quinoa, rolled oats, rye bread, wild rice; and whole wheat bread, cereal, crackers, pasta, and tortillas)

Foods to maintain a strategic distance from with diverticulitis

A few specialists prescribe maintaining a strategic distance from nuts, corn, and seeds, which are thought by some to plug Diverticular openings and cause diverticulitis, yet there is little confirmation to bolster this proposal. By and by, foods oftentimes prescribed to be maintained a strategic avoided from include:

- Popcorn
- Poppy seeds

- Sesame seeds

What about probiotics and diverticulitis or Diverticular disease?

Since irritation has been found at the edges of Diverticular, it has been theorized that colonic microscopic organisms might assume a part in the crack of Diverticular by advancing irritation. This has driven a few people to facilitate guess that changing the microbes in the colon may decrease irritation and burst and to propose treatment with probiotics and/or prebiotics; in any case, there is insufficient proof of an advantage of probiotics yet to suggest treatment with probiotics of patients with Diverticular disease.

What are the more genuine complexities of diverticulitis?

More genuine confusions of diverticulitis include:

> Collection of pus (abscess) in the pelvis where the diverticulum has ruptured
> Colonic hindrance because of broad irritation
> Generalized infection of the abdominal cavity (bacterial peritonitis)

> Bleeding into the colon

A diverticulum can break, and the microscopic organisms inside the colon can spread into the tissues encompassing the colon. This is then called diverticulitis. Constipation or or diarrhea additionally may happen with the aggravation. A gathering of discharge can create around the cracked diverticulum, prompting arrangement of a boil, ordinarily in the pelvis.

Aggravation encompassing the colon likewise can prompt colonic obstacle. Rarely, a diverticulum bursts openly into the stomach cavity bringing about an existence undermining disease called bacterial peritonitis. On uncommon events, the aroused diverticulum can dissolve into the urinary bladder, bringing about bladder contamination and going of intestinal gas in the pee. Much all the more infrequently the diverticulum can burst into the vagina.

Diverticular bleeding happens when the extending diverticulum dissolves into a vein inside the diverticulum. Rectal section of red, dim or maroon-shaded blood and clumps happen with no related stomach torment if there is no diverticulitis, yet bleeding into the colon additionally may happen amid a scene of diverticulitis. Blood from a diverticulum of the right colon may bring about the stool to end up dark in shading. Bleeding might be persistent or discontinuous, enduring a few days.

Patients with dynamic bleeding ordinarily are hospitalized for perception. Intravenous liquids are given to bolster the circulatory strain. Blood transfusions are fundamental for those with moderate to extreme blood loss. In an uncommon individual with lively and extreme bleeding, the pulse may drop, creating unsteadiness, stun, and loss of awareness. In many patients, bleeding stops suddenly and they are sent home following a few days in the healing center. Patients with relentless, extreme bleeding require surgical expulsion of the bleeding diverticulum albeit a few nonsurgical medications have been proposed.

How is diverticulitis and diverticulosis analyzed?

The signs and symptoms of diverticulitis are basic and sufficiently unmistakable that the nearness of diverticulitis is typically suspected. On the off chance that suspected, the analysis can be affirmed by an assortment of tests. Barium X-beams (barium bowel purges) can be performed to envision the colon. Diverticular are seen as barium filled pockets distending from the colon divider.

Direct perception of within the colon and the openings of the Diverticular should be possible with adaptable tubes embedded through the rectum and progressed into the colon. Either short tubes (sigmoidoscopes) or more tubes (colonoscopes) might be utilized to help with the finding and to prohibit different diseases that can imitate Diverticular disease.

In patients associated with having diverticulitis ultrasound and electronic tomography (CT) examinations of the stomach area and pelvis should be possible to identify irritation of the tissues encompassing the cracked diverticulum or accumulations of discharge

What home treatment or cures soothe diverticulitis symptoms?

Patients may have various scenes of Diverticular disease or diverticulitis, and might be hard to recognize the two. Milder scenes of torment might be dealt with at home with bed rest, prescriptions for torment and fit, and an unmistakable fluid diet. Patients ought to take their temperature as often as possible and push on their lower left guts where most Diverticular are found. At the principal indication of fever or expanding delicacy - indications of aggravation - a specialist ought to be counseled instantly for a conceivable visit to his office and/or the start of anti-infection agents; there is nothing as profitable as a physical examination by the specialist to settle on choices about further treatment or hospitalization.

What prescriptions treat diverticulitis and diverticulosis?

Most patients with diverticulosis have negligible or no symptoms, and don't require a particular treatment. A typical fiber diet is fitting to counteract blockage and maybe keep the arrangement of more Diverticular.

Patients with gentle symptoms of stomach pain because of strong fit in the range of the Diverticular may profit by hostile to uncontrollable medications, for example,

Chlordiazepoxide (Librax), dicyclomine (Bentyl),

Atropine, scopolamine, phenobarbital (Donnatal), and hyoscyamine (Levsin).

At the point when diverticulitis happens, anti-toxins for the most part are required. Oral anti-infection agents are adequate when symptoms are gentle. A few case of normally recommended anti-microbials include:

Ciprofloxacin (Cipro), metronidazole (Flagyl),

Cephalexin (Keflex) and doxycycline (Vibramycin).

What are different medications for diverticulitis?

Fluid or low fiber foods are informed during intense attacks with respect to diverticulitis. This is done to decrease the measure of material that goes through the colon, which in any event hypothetically, may irritate the diverticulitis. In extreme diverticulitis with high fever and pain, patients are hospitalized and given intravenous anti-infection agents. Surgery is required for patients with steady entrails obstacle, bleeding, or sore not reacting to antibiotics.

What is the surgical treatment for diverticulitis?

Diverticulitis that does not react to restorative treatment requires surgical mediation. Surgery normally includes drainage of any collections of discharge and resection (surgical evacuation) of the portion of the colon containing the Diverticular, as a rule the sigmoid colon. Surgical expulsion of the bleeding diverticulum likewise is important for those with determined bleeding. In patients requiring surgery to stop industrious bleeding, it is important to decide precisely where the bleeding is originating from keeping in mind the end goal to direct the specialist.

Now and then, Diverticular can disintegrate into the nearby urinary bladder, creating serious intermittent pee contamination and entry of gas amid pee. This circumstance additionally requires surgery.

Now and then, surgery might be proposed for patients with regular, repetitive attacks of diverticulitis prompting different courses of anti-toxins, hospitalizations, and days lost from work. During surgery, the objective is to evacuate all, or all, of the colon containing Diverticular so as to anticipate future scenes of diverticulitis. There are few long haul results of resection of the sigmoid colon for diverticulitis, and the surgery frequently should be possible laparoscopically, which limits post-operative pain and time for recuperation.

Chapter 2

To Know More about Diverticulitis

What is fiber?

What is fiber?

Fiber is a substance in foods that originates from plants. Fiber diminishes stool so it moves easily through the colon and is less demanding to pass. Solvent fiber disintegrates in water and is found in beans, organic product, and oat items. Insoluble fiber does not break down in water and is found in entire grain items and vegetables. Both sorts of fiber forestall stoppage. Obstruction is a condition in which a grown-up has less than three solid discharges a week or has defecations with stools that are hard, dry, and little, making them excruciating or hard to pass.

High-fiber foods likewise have numerous advantages in counteracting and controlling incessant maladies, for example, cardiovascular illness, stoutness, diabetes, and disease.

Who gets diverticulosis and Diverticular infection?

Diverticulosis turns out to be more normal as individual's age, especially in individuals more established than age 50.3 Some individuals with diverticulosis create diverticulitis, and the quantity of cases is expanding. In spite of the fact that Diverticular disease is for the most part thought to be a condition found in more seasoned grown-ups, it is turning out to be more regular in individuals more youthful than age 50, the greater part of whom are male.

What are the side effects of Diverticular infection?

Individuals with diverticulitis may have numerous side effects, the most widely recognized of which agony in the lower is left half of the stomach area. The torment is normally serious and goes ahead all of a sudden; however it can likewise be gentle and afterward decline more than a few days. The force of the agony can vacillate.

Diverticulitis may likewise bring about

- Fevers and chills

- Sickness or heaving
- An adjustment in gut propensities—blockage or the runs
- Diverticular seeping

  As a rule, individuals with Diverticular draining abruptly have a lot of red or maroon-hued blood in their stool.

Diverticular draining may likewise bring about

- Shortcoming
- Dazedness or discombobulating
- stomach cramping

How are diverticulosis and Diverticular illness analyzed?

Diverticulosis

Medicinal services suppliers regularly discover diverticulosis amid a normal x beam or a colonoscopy, a test used to peer inside the rectum and whole colon to screen for colon malignancy or polyps or to assess the wellspring of rectal dying.

Diverticular Sickness

In view of side effects and seriousness of disease, a man might be assessed and analyzed by an essential consideration doctor, a crisis division doctor, a specialist, or a gastroenterologist—a specialist who works in digestive diseases.

The medicinal services supplier will get some information about the individual's wellbeing, indications, inside propensities, eating regimen, and drugs, and will perform a physical exam, which may incorporate a rectal exam. A rectal exam is performed in the social insurance supplier's office; anesthesia is not required. To perform the exam, the human services supplier requests that the individual twist around a table or lie on one side while holding the knees near the mid-section. The medicinal services supplier slides a gloved, greased up finger into the rectum. The exam is utilized to check for torment, dying, or a blockage in the digestive system.

The social insurance supplier may plan one or a greater amount of the accompanying tests:

• **Blood test**. A blood test includes drawing a man's blood at a medicinal services supplier's office, a business office, or a healing facility and sending the example to a lab for examination. The blood test can demonstrate the nearness of irritation or paleness—a condition in which red platelets are less or littler than ordinary, which keeps the body's cells from getting enough oxygen.

• **Mechanized tomography (CT) examines.** A CT sweep of the colon is the most widely recognized test used to analyze Diverticular infection. CT filters utilize a mix of x beams and PC innovation to make three-dimensional (3–D) pictures. For a CT sweep, the individual might be given an answer for beverage and an infusion of an exceptional color, called contrast medium. CT checks require the individual to lie on a table that slides into a passage molded gadget where the x beams are taken. The technique is performed in an outpatient focus or a doctor's facility by a x-beam expert, and the pictures are deciphered by a radiologist—a specialist who represents considerable authority in medicinal imaging. Anesthesia is not required. CT sweeps can distinguish diverticulosis and affirm the analysis of diverticulitis.

• **Lower gastrointestinal (GI) arrangement.** A lower GI arrangement is an x-beam exam that is utilized to take a gander at the digestive organ. The test is performed at a doctor's facility or an outpatient focus by an x-beam specialist, and the pictures are translated by a radiologist. Anesthesia is not required.

The medicinal services supplier may give composed inside prep guidelines to take after at home before the test. The individual might be requested that take after a reasonable fluid eating regimen for 1 to 3 days before the strategy. A diuretic or douche might be utilized before the test. A purgative is pharmaceutical that extricates stool and expands solid discharges. A bowel purge includes flushing water or purgative into the rectum utilizing a unique squirt bottle. These drugs cause the runs, so the individual ought to remain nearby to a restroom amid the inside prep. For the test, the individual will lie on a table while the radiologist embeds an adaptable tube into the individual's rear-end. The colon is loaded with barium; making indications of Diverticular illness appear the entire more plainly on x beams. For a few days, hints of barium in the digestive organ can make stools be white or light hued. Douches and rehashed defecations may bring about butt-centric soreness. A medicinal services supplier will give particular directions about eating and drinking after the test. •

Colonoscopy. The test is performed at a healing facility or an outpatient focus by a gastroenterologist. Prior to the test, the individual's social insurance supplier will give composed entrails prep directions to take after at home. The individual may need to take after an unmistakable fluid eating routine for 1 to 3 days before the test.

The individual may likewise need to take intestinal medicines and bowel purges the night prior to the test. By and large, light anesthesia, and perhaps torment pharmaceutical, people groups unwind for the test.

The individual will lie on a table while the gastroenterologist embeds an adaptable tube into the rear-end. A little camera on the tube sends a video picture of the intestinal coating to a PC screen. The test can demonstrate diverticulosis and Diverticular sickness.

Cramping or bloating may happen amid the main hour after the test. Driving is not allowed for 24 hours after the test to permit the anesthesia time to wear off. Prior to the arrangement, individuals ought to make arrangements for a ride home. Full recuperation is normal by the following day, and individuals ought to have the capacity to do a reversal to their ordinary eating routine.

How are diverticulosis and Diverticular illness treated?

A medicinal services supplier may treat the side effects of diverticulosis with a high-fiber eating routine or fiber supplements, prescriptions, and conceivably probiotics. Treatment for Diverticular disease changes, contingent upon whether a man has diverticulitis or Diverticular dying.

Diverticulosis

High-fiber diet. Thinks about have demonstrated that a high-fiber eating regimen can avert Diverticular illness in individuals who as of now have diverticulosis.2 A social insurance supplier may prescribe a moderate increment in dietary fiber to minimize gas and stomach inconvenience. For more data about fiber-rich sustenance, see "Eating, Eating regimen, and Food."

Fiber supplements. A human services supplier may suggest taking a fiber item, for example, methylcellulose (Citrucel) or psyllium (Metamucil) one to three times each day. These items are accessible as powders, pills, or wafers and give 0.5 to 3.5 grams of fiber for every measurement. Fiber items ought to be brought with no less than 8 ounces of water.

Drugs. Various studies recommend the drug mesalazine (Asacol), given either consistently or in cycles, might be successful at decreasing stomach torment and GI manifestations of diverticulosis. Research has likewise demonstrated that consolidating mesalazine with the anti-infection rifaximin (Xifaxan) can be altogether more powerful than utilizing rifaximin alone to enhance a man's side effects and keep up times of abatement, which means being free of symptoms.

Probiotics. Albeit more research is required, probiotics may treat the side effects of diverticulosis, keep the onset of diverticulitis, and diminish the possibility of intermittent side effects. Probiotics are live microscopic organisms, similar to those ordinarily found in the GI tract. Probiotics can be found in dietary supplements—in containers, tablets, and powders—and in a few sustenance, for example, yogurt.

To guarantee facilitated and safe consideration, individuals ought to examine their utilization of correlative and option restorative works on, including their utilization of dietary supplements and probiotics, with their human services supplier.

Diverticular bleeding

Diverticular bleeding is uncommon. On the off chance that you have bleeding, it can be serious. In a few people, the bleeding may stop without anyone else and may not require treatment. Be that as it may, in the event that you have bleeding from your rectum—even a little sum—you ought to see a specialist immediately.

To discover the site of the bleeding and stop it, a specialist may play out a colonoscopy. Your specialist may likewise utilize an automated tomography (CT) check or an angiogram to discover the bleeding site. An angiogram is a unique sort of x-beam in which your specialist strings a dainty, adaptable tube through an extensive corridor, frequently from your crotch, to the bleeding region.

Colon resection

In the event that you're bleeding does not stop, a specialist may perform stomach surgery with a colon resection. In a colon resection, the specialist expels the influenced some portion of your colon and joins the rest of the closures of your colon together. You will get general anesthesia External NIH Link for this strategy.

Now and again, amid a colon resection, it may not be ok for the specialist to rejoin the finishes of your colon immediately. For this situation, the specialist plays out a provisional colostomy. A while later, in a brief moment surgery, the specialist rejoins the closures of your colon and shuts the opening in your stomach area.

Diverticulitis

Diverticulitis with gentle manifestations and no complexities more often than not requires a man to rest, take oral anti-infection agents, and be on a fluid eating routine for a timeframe. In the event that side effects ease following a couple days, the human services supplier will suggest steadily including strong sustenance once again into the eating regimen. Serious instances of diverticulitis with intense torment and intricacies will probably require a healing center remain.

Most instances of extreme diverticulitis are treated with intravenous (IV) anti-toxins and a couple days without food or beverage to help the colon rest. On the off chance that the period without sustenance or beverage is longer, the individual might be given parenteral food—a technique for giving an IV fluid food blend through an uncommon tube in the mid-section. The blend contains proteins, starches, fats, vitamins, and minerals.

What is the reason of diverticulitis and how are they treated?

Diverticulitis can assault abruptly and cause inconveniences, for example,

• **A sore**—an excruciating, swollen, pus-filled range simply outside the colon divider—brought about by disease

• **An aperture**—a little tear or opening in the Diverticular

• **Peritonitis**——inflammation of tissues inside the stomach area from discharge and stool that hole through a puncturing

- **A fistula**—an irregular section, or passage, between two organs, or between an organ and the outside of the body

- **Intestinal hindrance**—incomplete or all out blockage of development of sustenance or stool through the digestion tracts

These difficulties should be dealt with to keep them from deteriorating and bringing about genuine sickness. Now and again, surgery might be required.

Sore, puncturing, and peritonitis.

Anti-infection treatment of diverticulitis typically forestalls or treats a boil. On the off chance that the boil is substantial or does not clear up with anti-microbial, it might should be depleted. Subsequent to giving the individual desensitizing pharmaceutical, a radiologist embeds a needle through the skin to the canker and afterward depletes the liquid through a catheter. The technique is typically guided by a stomach ultrasound or a CT filter. Ultrasound utilizes a gadget, called a transducer that bobs sheltered, effortless sound waves off organs to make a picture of their structure.

A man with a puncturing for the most part needs surgery to repair the tear or opening. Here and there, a man needs surgery to evacuate a little part of the digestive system if the aperture can't be repaired.

A man with peritonitis might be to a great degree sick, with sickness, retching, fever, and serious stomach delicacy. This condition requires prompt surgery to clean the stomach hole and perhaps a colon resection at a later date after a course of anti-infection agents.

A blood transfusion might be required if the individual has lost a lot of blood. Without brief treatment, peritonitis can be deadly.

Fistula. Diverticulitis-related contamination may prompt one or more fistulas. Fistulas more often than not frame between the colon and the bladder, small digestive system, or skin. The most well-known sort of fistula happens between the colon and the bladder. Fistulas can be rectified with a colon resection and expulsion of the fistula.

Intestinal block. Diverticulitis related aggravation or scarring brought about by past irritation may prompt intestinal impediment. In the event that the digestive system is totally blocked, crisis surgery is important, with conceivable colon resection. Fractional blockage is not a crisis, so the surgery or different techniques to right it can be booked.

At the point when earnest surgery with colon resection is vital for diverticulitis, two methodologies might be required on the grounds that it is not protected to rejoin the colon immediately. Amid the colon resection, the specialist performs a brief colostomy, making an opening, or stoma, in the midriff. The end of the colon is associated with the opening to permit typical eating while recuperating happens. Stool is gathered in a pocket appended to the stoma on the stomach divider. In the second surgery, a while later, the specialist rejoins the finishes of the colon and shuts the stoma.

Eating, Eating routine, and Sustenance
The Dietary Rules for Americans

2010, suggests a dietary fiber admission of 14 grams for every 1,000 calories expended. Case in point, for a 2,000-calorie consume less calories, the fiber proposal is 28 grams for every day. The measure of fiber in a sustenance is recorded on the's food certainties name. A portion of the best wellsprings of fiber incorporate natural products; vegetables, especially boring ones; and entire grains. A social insurance supplier or dietitian can help a man figure out how to include all the more high-fiber sustenance into the eating regimen.

Which sustenance is high in fiber?

- Crisp products of the soil
- Wholegrain breads and grains
- Nuts and seeds
- Vegetables e.g. heated beans, lentils, kidney beans, soy beans

Low Irritant, High Fiber Diet for Diverticular Disease

Diverticular malady is the nearness of little "pockets" in the extensive entrails.

An entrails food which gets caught in the pockets may bring about agony and looseness of the bowels - this is called diverticulitis.

Changes to your eating routine can avert diverticulitis.

1.   Aim to take 8-10 measures of liquid for each day. Have a blend of beverages.

2.   Increase your admission of fiber from wholegrain grain foods, for example, wholegrain breakfast oats and whole meal bread.

3.   Foods named "Foods to attempt with alert" can influence some individuals.

Bring them step by step into your eating routine or stay away from totally in the event that you know they cause your manifestations.

	Foods to Take	Foods to Try With Caution
Vegetables :	Well-cooked mashed root vegetables, green vegetables e.g. cabbage, sprouts, spinach (no	Cucumber, radishes, whole tomatoes, peas, lentils, peppers, onions, sweet corn,

	Stalks), cauliflower, mushrooms, runner beans.	Bean sprouts. all kinds of beans, e.g. broad
	Lettuce, tomatoes (without skins & pips) E.g. tinned plum de-seeded tomatoes. Potatoes - all kinds without skin.	Beans, baked beans. Jacket potatoes.
Fruit:	Stewed, tinned or fresh, fruit skinned and Dipped. Fruit juice with no "stringy Bits".	Skins and pips of fruit. Dried fruit, e.g. currants, prunes, sultanas. Raspberries, strawberries,

		blackcurrants, blueberries, cherries, grapes, gooseberries, Rhubarb, coconut.
Meat and fish:	All	
Dairy Produce:	Milk, cheese, plain or flavored yoghurt, forage fraise, cream, butter, margarine, eggs, ice cream, Milk puddings.	Fruit yoghurts with pips e.g. Strawberry/raspberry.
Cereals:	Whole meal bread, whole meal flour, whole meal Biscuits e.g. digestive. Whole meal scones, whole meal cakes and	Granary bread. Cake/scones/biscuits Containing fruit.

	Pastries. Whole meal cereals, e.g. All Bran, Weetabix, Shredded Wheat, Porridge. Whole meal pasta, brown rice.	
Miscellaneous:	Sugar, honey, syrup, jelly, jam & marmalade without pips/seeds, bramble/fruit jelly, lemon Curd, chocolate, toffee, sweets, salt, pepper.	Fried foods. Marmalades/jams with seeds, skins and pips. Vinegar, highly seasoned & spiced foods e.g. curry, chili, chutney, pickles, nuts, peanut Butter.
Drinks:	Squash, tea,	Alcohol

	coffee, Ovaltine, Complain, Oxo, Bovril.	
Soup:	Cream or thickened soup.	Whole vegetable soup

Example Meal Plan

Breakfast

Fruit juice

Whole meal bread or toast with spread

Drink

Snack meal

Tuna sandwich using whole meal bread

Flavored yoghurt

Peeled fruit

Drink

Main meal

Cream soup

Meat, Potatoes, Vegetables (from list)

Gravy

Suitable fruit and custard

Glass of water or squash

Between meals and before bed

Drink and snack if required.

Additional drinks can be taken throughout day to achieve a total of 8-10 cups.

Chapter 3

Things you have to know

Some interesting new facts that have been developing about Diverticular disease have brought much of what is believed before into question. It has been discovered that there are many underlying facts that might just be precursors to this disease taking flight in your colon.

While inflammation is a part of an acute case of diverticulitis, it has recently been theorized that the inflammatory condition is most likely in place long before the diverticulitis becomes symptomatic. There were studies done that show a significant number of patients who developed diverticulitis later, first suffered from some other disease which involved inflammation of the colon like mesalazine. This is important because some drugs that people naturally take to reduce inflammation in most cases lead to more inflammation in the colon. This means that a person suffering from diverticulitis should avoid taking ibuprofen.

All patients can get tested to see if they are suffering from intestinal inflammation, a special stool test can tell you if this is the case or not. One of the most proactive things that a person can do to avoid an acute attack of diverticulitis is to make sure that they reduce any intestinal inflammation that exists.

One of the most natural things that can be done to reduce any inflammation in the intestines is to eat a healthy Paleo diet. This will allow you to avoid eating foods that are potentially irritating and inflammatory to the digestive tract such as whole grains and omega-6 fatty acids. A Paleo diet will also help keep the bacterial levels normal in the colon. This type of diet will focus on bone broths, well cooked vegetables, starchy tubers and fermented foods. These are all easily digested.

Stress Levels

Like in most things too much stress is going to have a negative impact on the diverticulitis that a patient is suffering. It is vital when trying to lower the level of intestinal inflammation of any kind to lower the stress a person experiences. Learning to manage stress is vital to maintaining a smooth digestive system. There are many options for great stress management.

All people face stress as a part of their lives, it is not the stress itself that causes problems like diverticulitis, it is a person's inability to deal with stress in a healthy way that does. Managing stress is really one of the most important skills that need to be managed in order to live a healthier and happier life each day. Taking away the pressure caused by stress is vital to your health and digestion.

Exercise is one of the most effective ways to manage stress. It allows all of the pressure to be worked off as you run, lift or bike your way to a healthier life. Cardio vascular exercise is the best because it provides a proper mind body connection that can end in stress. Exercise is also a real method of self-care that is always a good thing for your entire mental outlook. If you never take time for yourself and care for your health then it will be lost to diverticulitis or some other disease. The other added benefit of exercise is weight loss and it has been proven that the cases of diverticulitis occur less in patients who maintain a healthy weight.

Another great way to relieve stress is to start to develop an activity that teaches relaxation and calmness. These activities can include yoga, meditation or Tai chi. practicing these sorts of mental relaxation activities allow people to control and manage stress better and also let the stress go. It is another form of self-caring activity that will keep a person healthier and stop the development of Diverticular disease in your colon. Along with other techniques it is important to learn these mind body connections because they will stop inflammation in your digestive system and also the development of diverticulitis. Activities like meditation, yoga and the like are not difficult to do they just take a commitment and time to get them done.

Another great way to reduce inflammation in the digestive tract is to supplement your diet with healing and soothing demulcent herbs. Herbs are a natural remedy for stomach inflammation some of these are called marshmallow root and slippery elm. These can be found in some supplements and taken with water up to three times per day there is going to be a reduction in the inflammation in the colon and less of a chance that Diverticular disease will develop.

Maintain Bacterial Balance

One of the symptoms that are very common in diverticulitis patients is the intestinal bacterial overgrowth. That is too much development of harmful bacteria which leads to inflammation and damage to the entire system and makes all digestion less effective. Rifaximin is a drug that has been shown to affect this issue in a positive way by returning the bacterial balance to a more normal level. There are also simple foods that will do this as well, including some specialty yogurts.

Supplements That Help

A person suffering from diverticulitis may be able to find some significant relief by taking probiotic supplements. In combination with other treatments the probiotic nutrients can give a person a whole new lease on life. There are some great food choices that already include probiotics in them for example eating foods with kefir, kimchi or kombucha in them will naturally help reduce the effects of diverticulitis. Adding a supplement like Prescript Assist or VSL#3 is not a bad idea no matter where your health is currently at because it will improve your digestion and allow you to feel healthier each day.

Prebiotics are another option when it comes to correcting the level of good/bad bacteria in the digestive system. These are substances that are known to develop and nurture the growth and development of the positive forms of bacteria that will keep you healthy and manage your wellbeing. This is exactly what a person is looking for when they need to restore a healthy bacterial balance. One great perbiotic is fructose-oligosaccharide powder but consult a doctor or doctor to learn about more prebiotics that can help in solving a poor bacterial balance and help to stop diverticulitis before it begins.

Chapter 4

Eating Right is the Key

The colon is a vitally functioning organ in the human body and most people don't understand the function that it plays in the health of the body. It is the end of the digestive tract and runs around the entire stomach cavity. It is shaped like an inverted u and is a major part of the large intestine. The primary function of this apparatus is to maintain a balance of fluids in the body and to aid in the ability to absorb many vitamins and minerals and to remove waste from the body. When a person needs to get rid of wastes it goes to the colon which maintains our health and wellness. One of the reasons that nobody notices the function of the colon is that it works so well. It is only going to be noticed when it is not working to capacity.

When Diverticulitis hits this is the region that it affects. There is actually no real understanding of the causes of this disease but there is a lot of circumstantial evidence that a poor diet is the major culprit in causing this painful disease. Basically the symptoms of this disease can only be identified before an attack by a colonoscopy. Outside of that an attack of diverticulitis will occur when the pouches expand become inflamed and rupture. This will lead to some very difficult symptoms to deal with like diarrhea, blood in stool, fever, chills and vomiting. Unchecked this can lead to abscesses and fistulas or intestinal rupture, peritonitis and in extreme cases death.

The processed food of our fast food society seems to be one of the major culprits in feeding this disease. That is because Diverticular disease is virtually unheard of in underdeveloped nations where they eat nothing but fibrous natural foods. So not only is fast food a poor health choice for your health, it is also a poor choice for colon health as well. This is supported because when Eastern countries like Japan, China and Korea adopt more Western style foods the cases of diverticulitis increase significantly.

Now we get to the really important information of this chapter. The act of changing your diet can make it possible to wipe out Diverticular disease totally from the body. This will keep you in fine working order and allow for a happier and healthier working body system.

Get Your Fiber

Many doctors that have specialized in digestive tract illnesses have looked at what most people eat as a daily part of their diet and found that it is lacking in many of the essential nutrients that people should be eating for excellent digestive health. One of these ingredients is a diet that is much higher in fiber than is previously prescribed. One of the major contributors to the development of diverticulitis is that a person has difficulty in passing waste out of the colon through the rectum. A diet high in fiber will make this much easier and alleviate much of the problem. After the muscles in a person's colon spend years straining to perform their function due to a diet that is low in fiber there is a development of this issue. Particularly in the United States this can be seen. Doctors start to realize that the colon is becoming a bit stretched which makes it even more difficult to pass excrement from the body and the stool needs to be even bulkier to be moved out without difficulty.

There was a study done by the Journal of Nutrition that observed nearly 45,000 health professionals participating in a long term study. They learned that when a person ate a diet that was high in fiber they lowered the risk of

74

contracting Diverticular disease by somewhere in the neighborhood of 40%.

A high fiber diet presents a lot of other benefits as well. It fills your stomach easily and suppresses your appetite with can have a major assist in losing weight. Losing weight can help fight against developing Diverticular disease indirectly. Diverticular disease is much more likely to put a woman in the hospital if she is overweight or inactive. This is according to a study that was published in the American Journal of Gastroenterology.

It is recommended currently that 25 grams of fiber should be consumed by women each and every day. While men should eat even more fiber, being advised to try to consume about 38 grams of fiber in the daily diet. Even with these warnings the average American eats about 15 grams of fiber a woefully low portion. One of the best ways to augment your lack of fiber is to include foods that are high in fiber at every meal and also for snacks throughout the day.

Great sources of fiber for your diet include whole grains, oatmeal whole wheat bread, and barley. There are also some other great foods that you can dig into like lentils, fruits, vegetables and beans to give your diet a kick. One of the best snacking foods for a fiber input into your diet is to eat plenty of dried fruits which are a terrific source of fiber.

This type of eating plan is referred to as a whole foods diet because it includes a lot of foods that are not processed and treated with chemicals like white rice and white bread. Both of these are going to help cause diverticulitis rather than cure it. Eliminating the food that is bad for you is just as important as adding the food that is good for the body.

There are two types of fiber to consider soluble and insoluble. They are both an important part of a healthy diet but for different reasons. The insoluble fiber that is found in vegetable peels of fruit and seeds will add bulk to the stool in the colon and make it easier to pass reducing the wearing strain on the muscle. Soluble fiber is the other kind that a body needs and it comes from foods like oatmeal, barley, and many fresh fruits like apples. This adds to the moisture located in the stool and that makes it easier to pass through the colon and reduces the strain.

Nuts

Many old fashioned doctors tell their patients to avoid eating nuts, seeds or popcorn if a patient is suffering from diverticulitis. They have a fear that these course foods will get stuck in the Diverticular and cause bleeding or in the worst case infection. However it seems that this recommendation is not supported by any evidence whatsoever. In fact, it seems that these foods are healthy snacks and provide an excellent source of fiber to keep a person healthy and functioning well. These are easy to get and snack on foods that should not be ignored.

Some Eating Tips

Although most Americans love to eat meat, there is a report out that states that vegetarians are at a risk of 31% lower to develop diverticulitis than a meat eater. This is based on a study that involved over 47,000 candidates of both men and women. Many contribute this improvement to the higher level of fiber in the vegetarian diet. Many also suggest that the wall of the colon is negatively impacted by the high concentrations of bacteria that eating a meat heavy diet introduce.

Drink More Fluids

It seems a simple solution but it is an effective one. Drinking more fluids can help a high fiber diet be moved even easier through the digestive process with fewer chances of obstructions developing. Keeping the fluid intake into a normal level is all that is needed. There doesn't seem to be much of a benefit for drinking excessive liquids during the day. Look to drink as many non-calorie beverages as you can with your diet each day that means no limits to water or tea.

Bacteria Problems

The colon is a mysterious place because it has a lot of bacteria living there to assist in the process of digestion. The problem is that a balance needs to be maintained inside of the colon in order for a person to be able to digest food in the most efficient manner possible. Some foods that can assist in balancing out the bacteria are miso and yogurt because they are both high in probiotics which can definitely help in defeating Diverticular disease in the colon.

It was learned in a study that a person who was suffering from the pain of diverticulitis was able to take a probiotic supplement along with a diet high in fiber and this significantly relieved the pain and bloating being felt in the abdomen. It is worth noting that there is no concrete evidence written in stone that the bacteria in fermented foods, like yogurt, can have a measurable impact on the bacteria in the colon or not. This is especially true if the diet is lacking in fiber.

Chapter 5

What to Expect with Diverticulitis

It is important to remember that having diverticulitis does not mean that there are going to be any symptoms visible for a person to observe. Many live blissfully unaware of their condition until they have an attack and then that painful uncomfortable situation will need to be treated by a doctor. One of the simple cures is with antibiotics but there are more serious cases that need to be handled with surgery.

Again we know that if you are suffering from diverticulitis, a liquid diet may be prescribed by your doctor as a part of your treatment. This will give the colon a chance to heal and recover without having to perform the task that it was designed for.

This type of liquid diet should include water, fruit juices, broth, ice pops and tea. Very slowly the patient can start to ease back into eating solid foods. However they really need to stop neglecting the fiber at this point and start to eat high fiber foods. Because of the medical condition the colon might have difficulty at first passing high fiber foods very well so your doctor will most likely prescribe foods that are lower in fiber to begin with. These include eggs, fish, poultry and all dairy products as well. Remember the more fiber that is present in the diet the more bulk there will be in the stool and that will reduce the pressure on the colon to perform its job.

There have been studies done that demonstrate quite clearly that fiber rich foods can help control the symptoms that diverticulitis brings to the table. Again it is urged that you try to eat at least 25-35 grams of fiber each and every day. The following great foods are just full with fiber and should be included in your diet.

> Whole grain breads, cereals and pastas

> Beans of many kinds including black beans and kidney beans

> All fresh fruits like prunes, pears and apples

> All fresh vegetables including spinach, potatoes, squash and peas

It can be difficult at first to design your own diet but there are many dieticians and medical professionals that can help in designing a healthy diet that is just chock full of delicious fiber. They may also recommend that a patient takes a fiber supplement as a part of a nutritious diet one to three times a day.

Some people may experience constipation with a high fiber diet but that can be avoided by simply focusing on drinking more fluids throughout your day.

Foods to Avoid

Of course there are going to be some foods that simply must be avoided when a person is suffering from diverticulitis.

Chapter 6

Some Ideas for Colon Health

So now that we have a handle on what diverticulitis is and what we should eat and not eat when it comes to combating this disease there should be a guide to refer to on a regular basis so that we can maintain a healthy colon and avoid diverticulitis in the easiest manner possible. In the case of this digestive trouble an ounce of prevention is worth a pound of cure and it takes very little knowledge and action to make sure that Diverticular disease is avoided totally. Here are some helpful hints and reminders to consider as your look for a healthy lifestyle.

Fiber

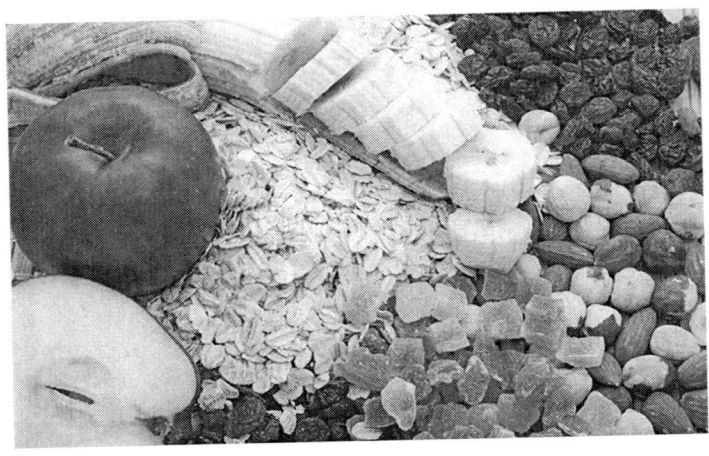

Eat a diet that is high in fiber. Of course we have made this point before but it is worth repeating. Eating more vegetables, whole grains, fruits and legumes can improve the health of your colon immensely. Having a high percentage of fiber in your diet helps waste move through your digestive tract and reduces the stress on the muscles of the colon as they are trying to discharge them. Diverticulitis will result when there is continual excess stress placed on the muscles of the colon to do their job. Fiber will also help in maintaining a healthy weight as well.

All types of Fiber

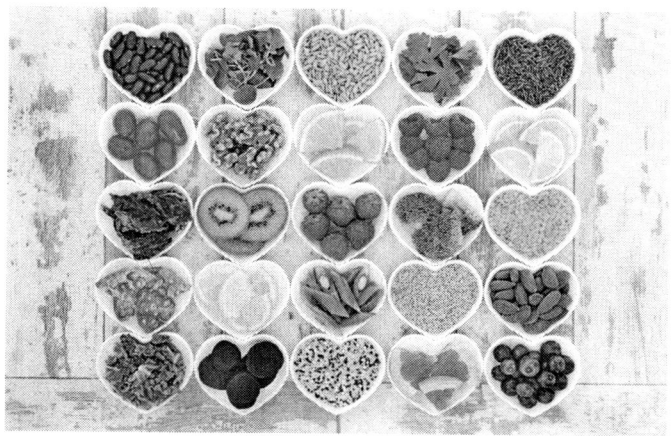

Make sure that both soluble and insoluble fiber is a part of your diet. That is important because they both affect your digestive system in different and positive ways. The soluble fiber attracts more moisture and water and that will allow for the easier passage of waste through the colon. Sources of soluble fiber are wheat bran, nuts, seeds and legumes. They can prevent soft stools from becoming too watery and this difficult to pass. The insoluble fiber is the classic roughage that can't be digested by the body but adds bulk to stools and makes them easier to expel.

Avoid Fatty Foods

Stay away for foods high in fat. It is no secret that foods that are high in fat tend to slow down the digestion process and can lead to episodes of constipation. This is not healthy for the colon because it causes undue stress on the muscles and can cause long term damage to them. It is also much easier to maintain a healthy weight if the foods that are high in fat are avoided.

Lean Meats

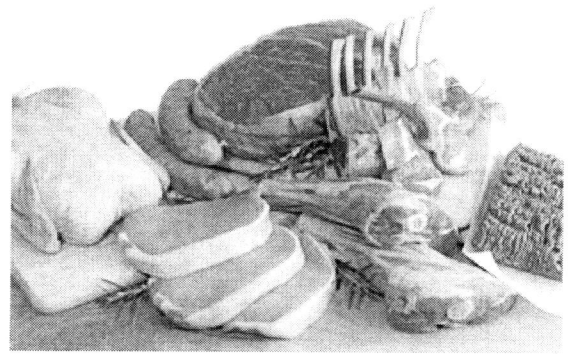

Eating meat is probably not going to be an option for many people because it has become such a part of our diets but the type of meat can be managed. Only eat the leanest mests when possible. Meats that have an excess of fatty tissue in them are not healthy for the digestion and they can introduce too much of the unhealthy kinds of bacteria in the colon, a perceived cause of diverticulitis. Some smart meats to eat are skinless poultry, pork loin and select lean cuts of steak.

Probiotics

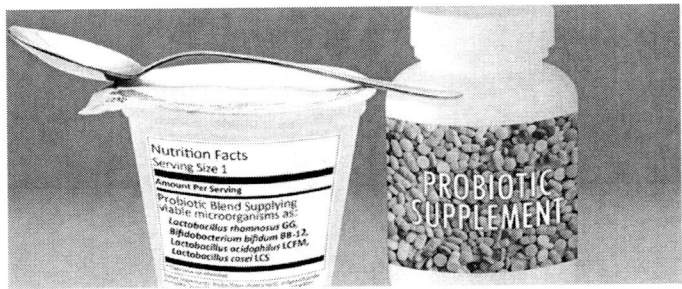

It is important to make sure probiotics are in your diet. Probiotics will add healthy bacteria to the digestive system and make the colon work smoother and more efficiently which will allow for less development of Diverticular disease. Probiotics enhance the ability of the body to take the nutrients from food, breakdown lactose and even help improve the immune system of the body. Low fat yogurt or kefirs are a great source of probiotics for people to consume in order to avoid Diverticular disease.

Eat regularly

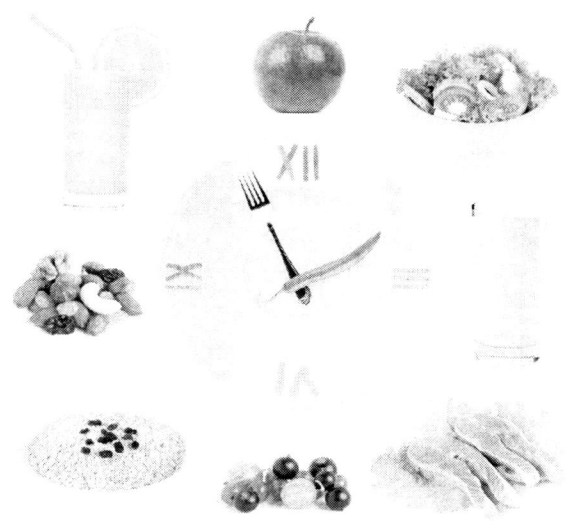

It is important to develop a normal eating schedule each day. It is believed that eating all of your snacks and meals at the same time each day will allow for your digestive system and colon to work in a more regular fashion and that will keep your colon in great shape and avoid the development of Diverticular disease. Make a goal to have your main three meals at about the same time each day along with any snacks. Most people are creatures of habit and this can become easy to do.

Drink Plenty

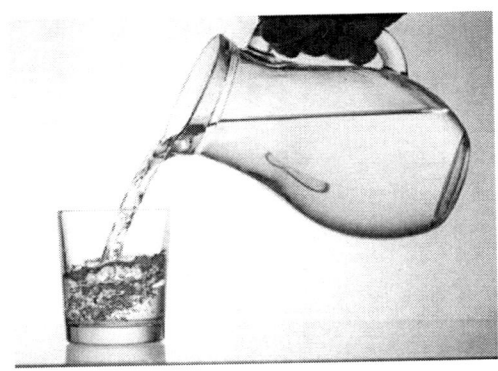

Like almost all things in our health, drinking plenty of water makes our bodies run better and more efficiently. Having the proper hydration will allow your digestive system to process food quicker and easier and move it through the digestive tract to the colon and be passed out of the body easier. This reduces stress on the muscles of the colon and allows for less of a chance of developing diverticulitis.

Avoid hurting yourself

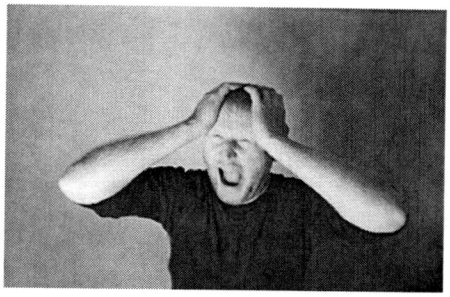

Sometimes many people are their own worst enemies when it comes to health and if you smoke or drink then you are increasing the chances that you will develop Diverticular disease. Smoking destroys the colon's ability to pass stools out of the body easily and that causes Diverticular disease. Alcohol leads to dehydration and that will make it difficult to process foods in the colon as well creating undue stress on the muscles which causes diverticulitis. If you smoke or drink alcohol than stop immediately. It is good for the best colon health.

Stress management

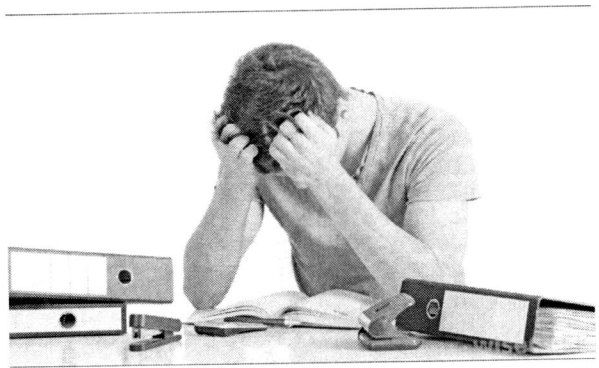

As we mentioned before anxiety and stress can cause some problems in the digestive tract. Make sure that you adopt a positive stress management plan on a regular basis.

Remember that what you eat and your behaviors are going to be completely intertwined with the chances that you develop diverticulitis. So referring to this chart and making positive changes can help you develop a healthier colon and allow you to experience a higher quality of life.

Chapter 7

The Recap

Diverticulitis is a disease that affects many people in the United States today. As a person gets older the risk of suffering from the disease is going to rise. There are many choices that we make in our diet which will either control or cause Diverticular disease to develop. People can go through much of their lives with no symptoms showing but still be developing this disease. Once the disease shows itself then it is very dangerous and painful.

Even after all of the symptoms have been shown a person can overcome this ravages of diverticulitis by changing their diet to one that is far healthier and consists of fiber. There is a lot of misinformation on the market today that is outdated and untrue. Some older literature suggests that people should avoid nuts or popcorn because it may irritate the Diverticular disease but recent studies have shown that this is not the case. In fact, these foods can actually help pass stools faster and easier from the colon and that will allow for less stress on the muscles of the colon.

Chapter 8

A Picture Guide to Diverticulitis

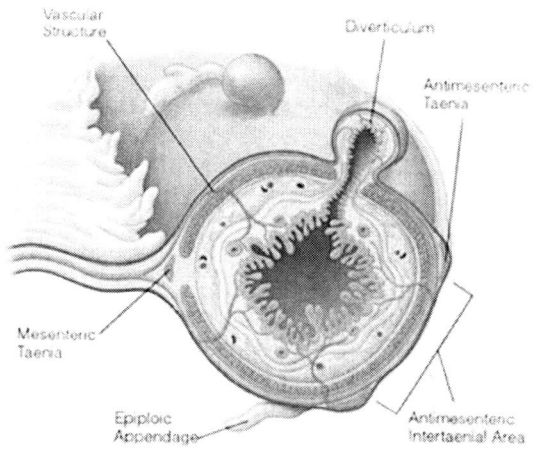

What Are a Diverticulum and Diverticular?

A diverticulum is a protruding pocket or sac that can frame on interior organs. In this slide show we will examine colonic Diverticular, which are protruding sacs that push outward on the colon divider. Diverticular can happen any place in the colon, yet most ordinarily frame close to the end of the colon on the left side (sigmoid colon).

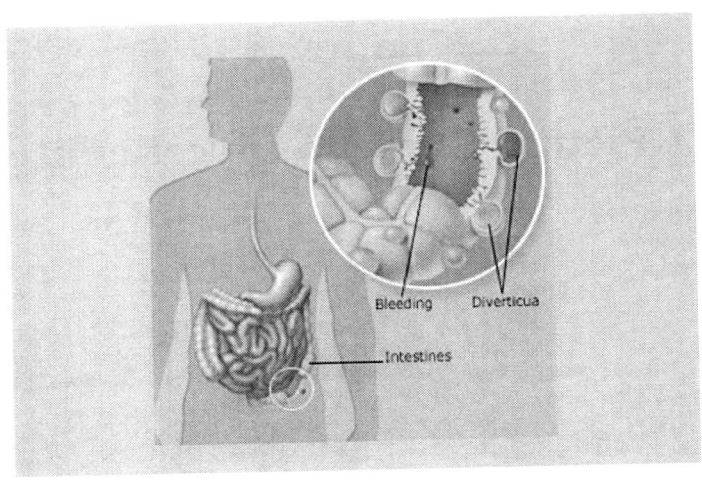

Bleeding Diverticua

Intestines

What Is Diverticulitis?

On the off chance that a diverticulum gets to be aroused or infected or the region around the diverticulum is swollen, it is called diverticulitis. On the off chance that the irritation or disease gets to be sufficiently extreme, the diverticulum can burst, spreading microorganisms from the colon to the encompassing tissues, bringing on a contamination called peritonitis, or framing a pocket of contamination called a boil.

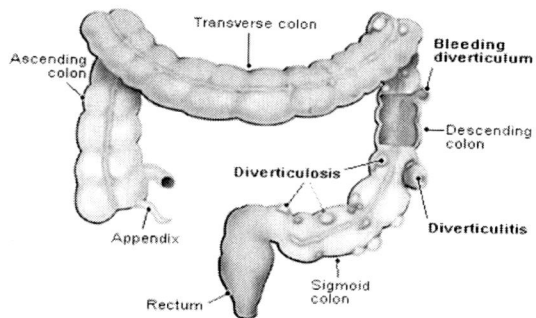

What Is Diverticulosis?

At the point when a patient has Diverticular (swelling sacs) in the colon this is called Diverticulitis or Diverticular disease.

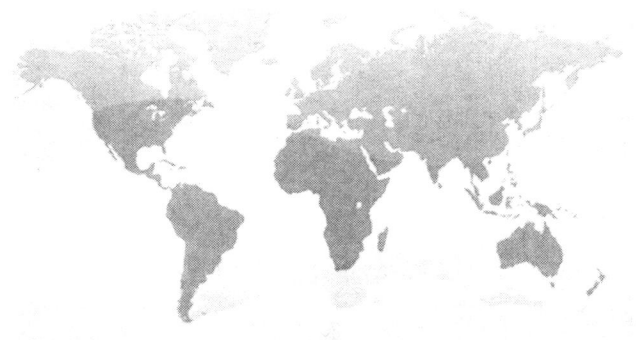

How Common Is Diverticular Disease?

Diverticular disease is most normal in industrialized nations where diets are lower in fiber and higher in handled sugars. The U.S., England, and Australia, see a bigger number of instances of Diverticular disease than spots, for example, Asia or Africa, where diets are wealthier in fiber.

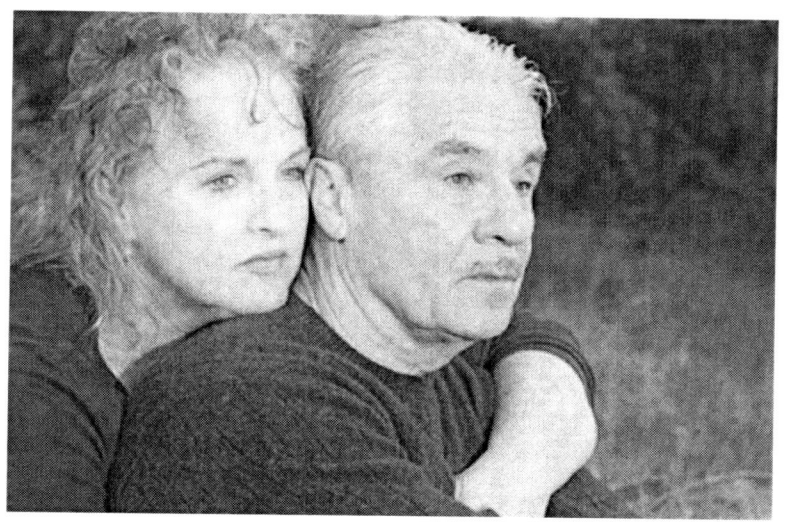

Who Gets Diverticular Disease?

In the U.S., Diverticular disease is found in more than half of individuals beyond 60 years old. Around 10%-25% of individuals with Diverticular disease will encounter an irritation of a diverticulum, bringing about contamination (diverticulitis).

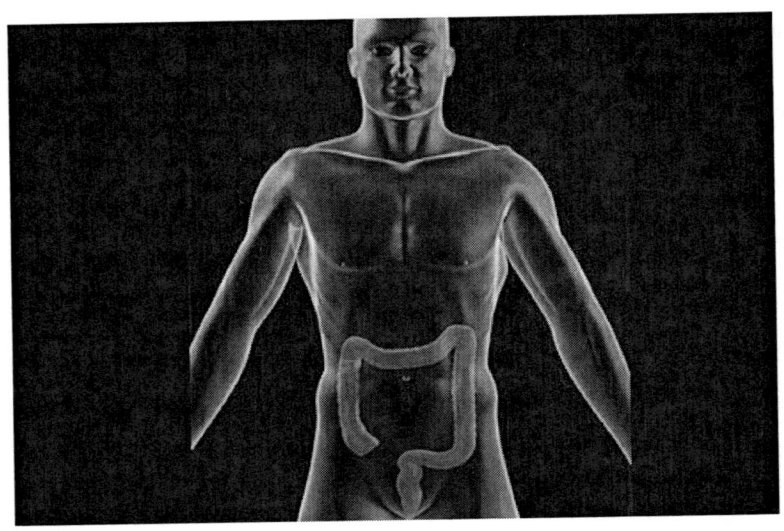

What Causes Diverticular?

It is trusted Diverticular structure when there is expanded weight in the colon. This expanded weight has a few conceivable causes. Diets low in fiber cause hard stool and slower "transit time" (the time it takes for stool to go) through the colon, expanding weight. Moreover, rehashed straining during solid discharges likewise builds weight. A few meds, for example, pulse drugs, "water pills" (diuretics), and opiate torment relievers, can expand blockage and expansion weight in the colon. Any of these reasons for expanded weight can prompt the development of Diverticular.

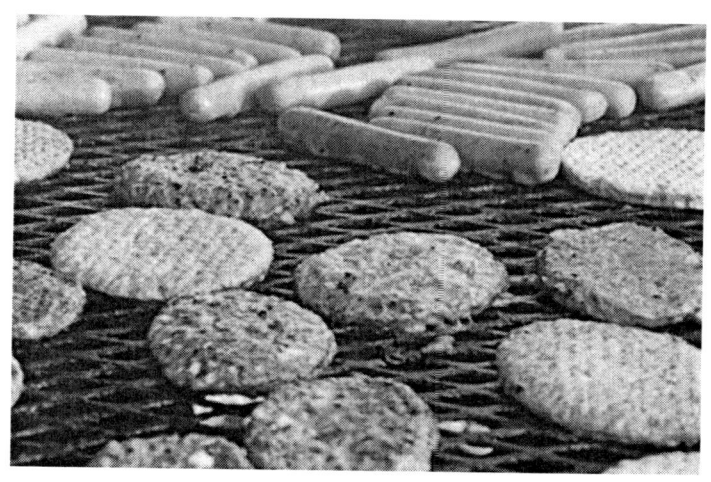

How Does Diet Contribute To Diverticulosis?

Diets low in fiber cause stool to be harder, and can prompt clogging. Obstruction can bring about rehashed straining during solid discharges, and can build the weight in the colon, which can prompt the development of Diverticular. Diets higher in fiber can anticipate stoppage and straining and may diminish the danger for Diverticular development.

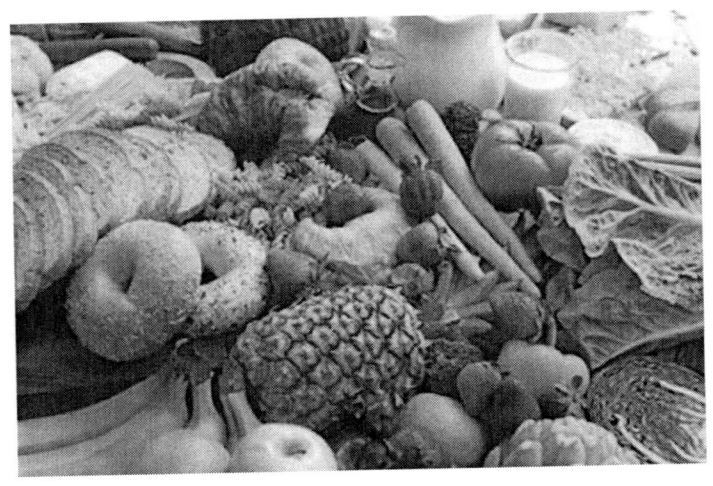

What Foods Are High In Fiber?

There are two sorts of dietary fiber expected to keep stool delicate and to avoid obstruction. Solvent fiber breaks up in water and structures a delicate gel-like substance in the digestive tract. Insoluble fiber goes through the digestive tract almost unaltered and can have a diuretic impact, stooling to pass. Great wellsprings of fiber incorporate leafy foods, entire grains, and vegetables, for example, beans or lentils.

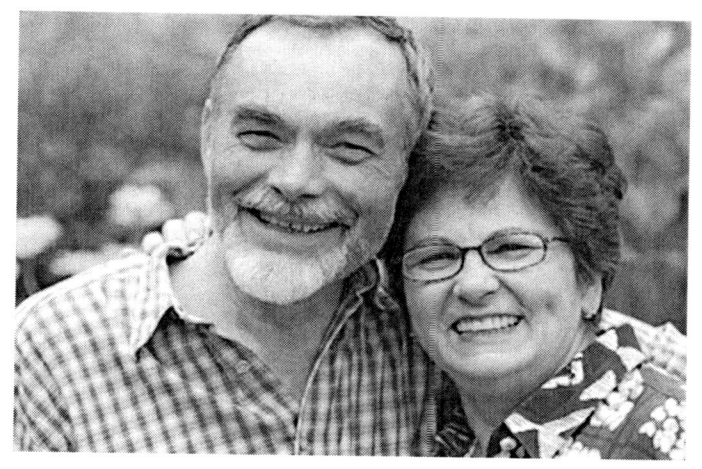

What Are the Most Common Symptoms of Diverticular Disease?

Numerous patients with Diverticular disease encounter no symptoms. Around 20% of patients will encounter a few symptoms that may incorporate stomach cramping, bloating, stomach swelling, rectal pain, and diarrhea.

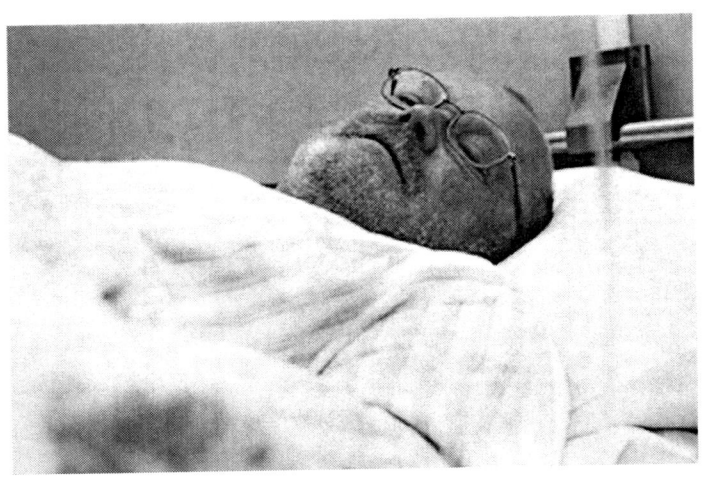

What Are the Serious Symptoms and Complications of Diverticulitis?

Sometimes, patients may encounter extreme difficulties of Diverticular disease, including:

> Extreme diverticulitis (contamination of the diverticulum)
> A collection of pus in the pelvis (a boil) because of burst of the diverticulum
> Generalized infection of the stomach hole (bacterial peritonitis)
> Colonic check
> Bleeding into the colon

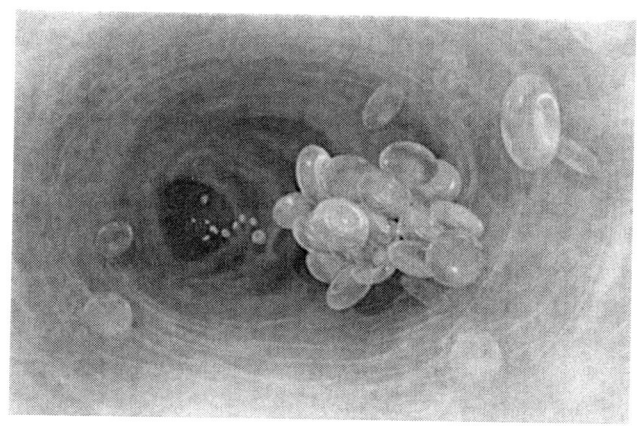

What Causes Bleeding With Diverticular Disease?

At the point when the aggravation of the diverticulum dissolves into a vein at the base of the diverticulum (sac) this can prompt Diverticular bleeding which can bring about red, dim, or maroon-hued blood and clumps to be passed when the patient has a solid discharge? The patient could conceivably encounter stomach pain. The bleeding may happen on and off, or keep going for a few days persistently. In the event that there is dynamic bleeding, the patient is generally hospitalized. In the event that the bleeding is extreme it might oblige treatment to stop the bleeding or surgery to remove the Diverticular.

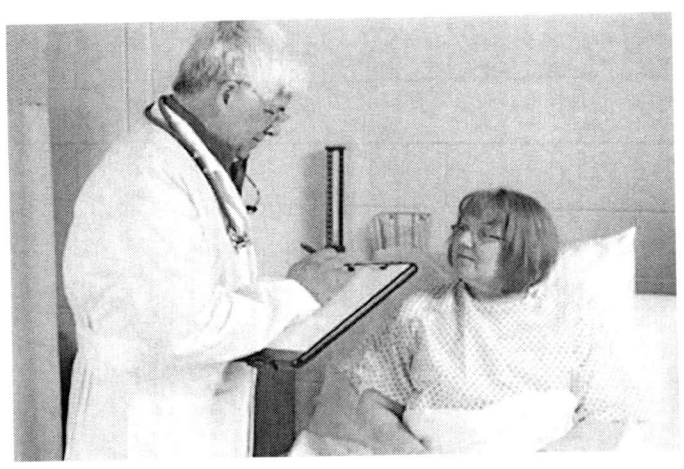

When Should I Call the Doctor?

See your specialist on the off chance that you have any of the accompanying symptoms and have been determined previously to have Diverticular disease:

Stomach pain Fever Diarrhea Vomiting Rectal bleeding (regardless of the possibility that it stops all alone) – this might be an indication of diverticulosis, diverticulitis, or different genuine conditions.

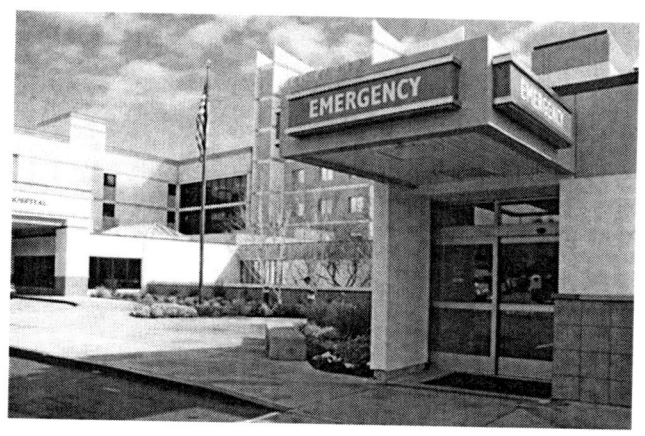

When Should I Go to the Emergency Department?

Go to a crisis division instantly on the off chance that you have known Diverticular or past episodes of diverticulitis and you encounter any of the accompanying symptoms:

- ➢ Serious stomach torment
- ➢ Steady fever going with stomach torment
- ➢ Serious spewing
- ➢ Steady obstruction with stomach swelling or bloating
- ➢ Serious torment or different symptoms you beforehand experienced during a session with diverticulitis

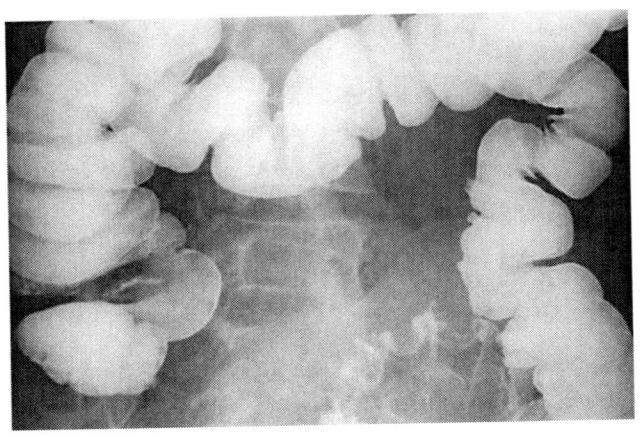

How Is Diverticulitis Diagnosed?

Diverticular are analyzed by sigmoidoscopy or colonoscopy, which are extensions with cameras used to glimpse inside the colon. Diverticular can likewise be determined to have a CT sweep of the belly and pelvis or a barium X-beam (barium bowel purge). During an intense erupt of diverticulitis a CT sweep might be utilized to analyze the degree of the contamination.

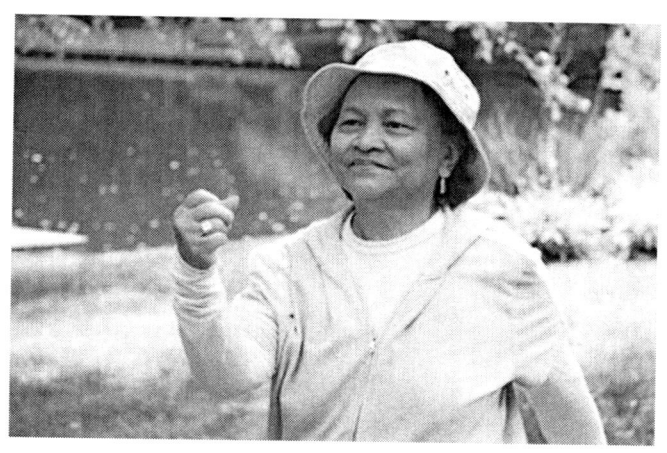

What Is the Treatment For a Patient With Diverticular Disease With Minimum or No Symptoms?

While numerous patients with Diverticular disease have few to no symptoms, a high fiber diet and fiber supplements are prescribed to avoid clogging and the development of extra Diverticular.

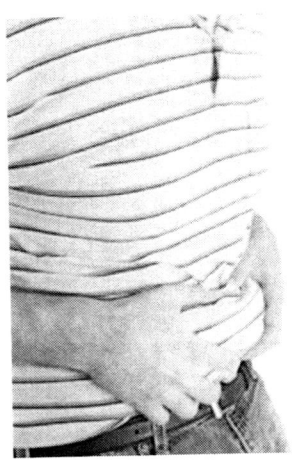

What Is the Medical Treatment For Mild Abdominal Pain Due To Diverticular Disease?

There are a few meds that can regard gentle symptoms, for example, stomach torment because of muscle fit. Antispasmodic drugs include:

> chlordiazepoxide (Librax)
> dicyclomine (Bentyl)
> hyoscyamine (Levsin)
> atropine, scopolamine, phenobarbital, hyoscyamine (Donnatal)
> diphenoxylate and atropine (Lomotil)

In the past specialists advised patients to avoid corn, nuts, and seeds they thought may get to be stopped in one of the

Diverticular and cause confusions, in any case, there is no confirmation these foods bring on a specific issues. Counsel your specialist in the event that you have concerns.

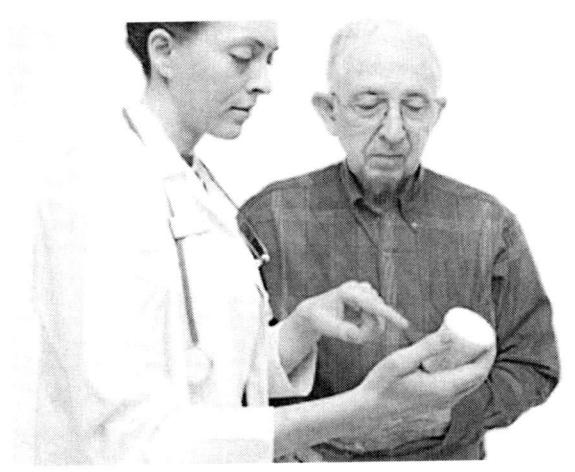

Are Antibiotics Used In the Treatment Of Diverticulitis?

In the event that you create diverticulitis (disease) because of an inflamed Diverticular, antibiotics might be recommended for gentle symptoms, including:

➤ ciprofloxacin (Cipro)

➤ levofloxacin (Levaquin)

➤ amoxicillin/clavulanic acid (Augmentin)

➤ metronidazole (Flagyl)

➤ doxycycline (Vibramycin)

In the event that you are encountering an intense assault of diverticulitis you might be encouraged to expend a fluid diet and low fiber foods.

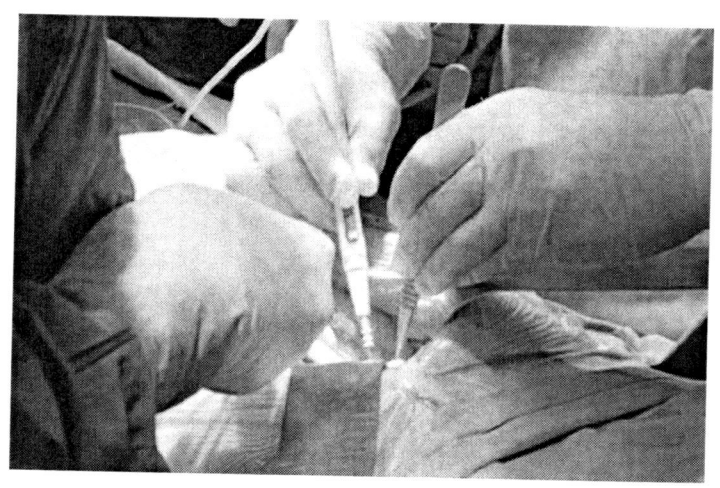

When Is Surgery Necessary For a Patient With Diverticulitis?

If diverticulitis does not react to therapeutic treatment, surgery might be required. This generally comprises of depleting any collections of discharge and surgically expelling the fragment of the colon where the Diverticular are found (as a rule the sigmoid colon). Industrious bleeding Diverticular require surgical evacuation. Surgery is likewise fundamental in situations where the Diverticular disintegrate into different organs, for example, the neighboring bladder (colovesical fistula), creating serious repetitive pee contaminations and section of gas during pee.

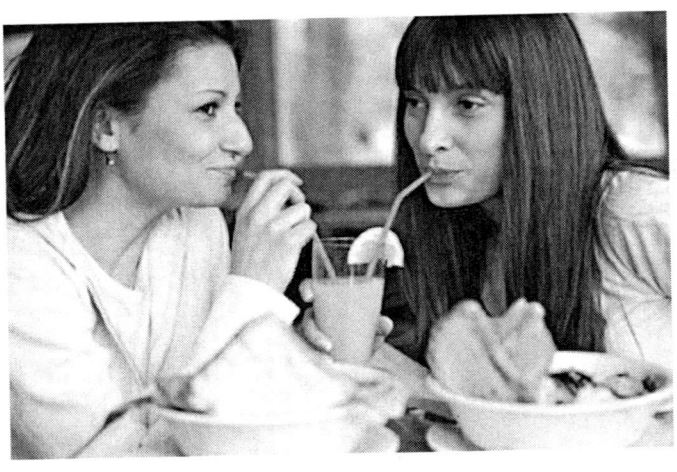

Can Diverticular Disease Be Prevented?

Diverticular are lasting once formed and must be expelled surgically. There is at present no treatment to forestall Diverticular disease. Be that as it may, diets high in fiber are prescribed to expand stool mass and forestall blockage, which decreases weight in the colon and may keep more Diverticular from framing, or worsening of the condition.

Conclusion

Much obliged to you again to download this book!

I trust this book could help you to comprehension diverticulitis.

At last, in the event that you delighted in this book, please take an ideal opportunity to share your musings and post an audit on Amazon. It'd be significantly refreshing!

Much obliged to you and good fortunes!

CPSIA information can be obtained
at www.ICGtesting.com
Printed in the USA
FFOW01n1311051216
30100FF